SCIENTIFIC HEALING

With Foods, Minerals and Colors

SCIENTIFIC HEALING

With Foods, Minerals and Colors

Ariel Gordon

PILGRIMS

PILGRIMS PUBLISHING

Varanasi • Kathmandu

SCIENTIFIC HEALING

By Ariel Gordon

Published by
PILGRIMS PUBLISHING

An imprint of
PILGRIMS BOOK HOUSE
B 27/98 A-8, Nawabganj Road
Durga Kund
Varanasi, India 221010
Tel: 91-542-314060, 312496
Fax: 91-542-314059
E-mail: pilgrims@satyam.net.in

Distributed in India by
BOOK FAITH INDIA
414-416 Express Tower
Azadpur Commercial Complex
New Delhi-110033, India
Tel: 91-11-713-2459
Fax: 91-11-724-9674
E-mail: pilgrim@del2.vsnl.net.in

Distributed in Nepal by
PILGRIMS BOOK HOUSE
P.O Box 3872
Kathmandu, Nepal
Tel: 977-1-424942
Fax: 977-1-424943
E-mail: pilgrims@wlink.com.np

First published in Santa Barbara by
J.F. Rowyn Press

ISBN 81-7769-017-5

Edited by C.N. Burchett
Layout by Hom KC
Cover design by Sasya

Printed in India

Contents

Introduction to the New Edition

Remembering the psychedelic light shows of the late sixties and the brightness of colors and the meaning they added to youth, this book is a refreshing return to nature in the age of chemical existence. Fresh vegetables, fresh air, pure colors are almost simply a memory now.

How we marvel at the heroes of bygone ages wielding swords and maces which ordinary men can hardly lift today, simply thinking these are only tales blown up or created in the minds of the story tellers. How we laugh behind our cuffs as old men ramble on about their good old days and how the food they ate then tasted like the nectar of the gods in comparison to the fare we get today. The young folk laugh to themselves as they gobble up greasy hamburgers or pieces of pizza hardly noticing the flavors as they greedily fill their stomachs to the full.

Now Ariel Gordon presents us with a drug free, chemical free regime with which to heal the sores of abuse which we have loaded upon our bodies. He gives us the keys to nature's garden from where we may heal our diseased souls upon the color and freshness which she provides. Mother nature has never forgotten her prodigals who have always tried to force their wanton changes upon their benefactor.

Learn how to diet without pills and appliances, cure this ailing body with the purity which nature offers still. Go back to your roots and learn what our fathers learn before us.

Maintain a balanced diet and enjoy the benefits of a healthy body. This is the message given by the author, which I am sure, all right thinking people would wish to follow.

Introduction

The acquisition of a radiantly healthy body and an enlightened mind is the greatest of human accomplishments. HEALTH is the condition of a true life: the result and sign of HEALTH is HAPPINESS. Unhappiness of every kind is the result of disease, whether of the body or the mind. Sorrow is just as much the effect of disease as pain. One is the outcry of a sick organism, the other of a wounded spirit.

During recent years many radical changes have been made in the realm of healing. Progressive physicians everywhere are devoting their attention more and more to NATURAL THERAPY, and cures are being performed now that have been impossible with the old Drug System.

THE PURPOSE of this work is to disseminate the findings of Science, in the realm of

DRUGLESS THERAPY, knowing that NATURE is the PERFECT DOCTOR.

Yours for successful living,
ARIEL GORDON, *Colourist-Dietitian.*

Part I

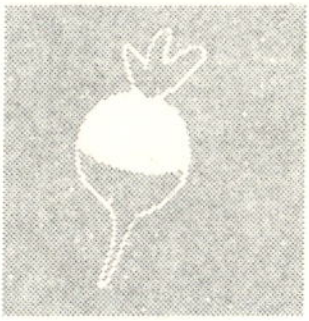

Nutrition

Our deportment, character and mental processes are regulated largely according to our nutrition. "Tell me what a man eats and I will tell you what he is," is a maxim which is self-evident. As we are made and remade of what we eat and drink, it is very important the HEALTH SEEKER understands the virtue of Proper Nutrition. Food will kill or cure according to its selection and use. The following information is supplied from the greatest dietetic authorities of the world.

Foods are divided into four classes: FATS, CARBOHYDRATES, PROTEINS, and FOOD SALTS.

The best FAT foods are butter, cream, olive and vegetable oils, and the fats of oils and nuts.

The CARBOHYDRATES include starches and the various sugars. The best sugars are raw brown sugar, honey and maple sugar; these should be used in preference to the ordinary refined white sugar which is deficient in natural minerals and is consequently acid producing. The starches are derived principally from vegetables and cereals.

PROTEIN is the body building and repair food. The best protein foods are eggs, cheese, milk, nuts, legumes (peas, beans, lentils, peanuts), cereals and certain kinds of vegetables. It may be asked, what is the protein value of meat? Recent experiments have proven that meat is inferior to the above mentioned foods, especially raw certified milk. However, when eaten in proper combination, by persons of good digestive systems, flesh foods may be eaten with benefit.

FOOD SALTS are so-called mineral substances found in natural foods, such as IRON and LIME, etc. These are essential elements of the tissues and a deficiency of any of the mineral salts is always disastrous to the health. Because these salts are so little understood, and due to their prime importance to HEALTH, we supply a complete list of these salts and the foods in which they are to be found in greatest abundance. The following data is supplied from the most authoritative sources in BIOCHEMISTRY.

1.CALCIUM

Calcium is required by the bones and teeth for hardness. Necessary for the muscles, heart, lungs, tissues, intestinal walls, arterial walls and other organs for strength. Obesity, chronic tiredness, consumption, flabby skin, low blood pressure, heart weakness, decaying teeth are often caused from CALCIUM DEFICIENCY. Bleeding from open wounds is difficult to stop where there is a lack of this element.

CALCIUM (Muscle) FOODS

Lemons	Raw Cabbage	Milk
Oranges	Citron	Dates
Bran	Tomatoes	Goat's Milk
Apricots	Halibut	Lettuce
All Fish	Limes	Swiss Cheese
Figs	Roquefort Cheese	Rhubarb
Spinach		

2. PHOSPHOROUS

Phosphorous is an element which electrifies and magnetizes the brain and nerves, improves the memory, makes one idealistic and intuitive. Use the juice of oranges with raw egg yolk, with or without honey, daily, between meals to train the brain cells to assimilate more phosphorus.

PHOSPHORUS (Brain) FOODS

Milk	Egg Yolk	Walnuts
Barley	Oats	Rye
Dates	Lentils	Prunes
Oranges	Bran	Beechnuts
Cabbage	Whole Wheat	All Fish
Peas		(Sea water)

3. SULPHUR

Sulphur produces energy and color stimulates blood circulation-corrects tendency to chronic tiredness and cold extremities. Sulphur improves the color of the hair and skin, and is a blood purifier. (Most of the sulphur foods are best eaten raw).

SULPHUR (Energy) FOODS

Figs & Dates	Carrots	Cauliflower
Radishes	Coconuts	Chestnuts
Turnips	Potatoes	Onions
Cucumbers	Almonds	Brussels Sprouts
Kohlrabi	Cabbage	Mustard
	Horse-radish	

4. IRON

Iron is the magnetizing element of the human machine. Iron is necessary to keep the blood red and magnetic. It is indispensable in the cure of anemia, a very devitalizing disease. Anemic persons should use plenty of orange juice and raw egg yolk daily, and an abundance or fresh air to oxidize the blood, as well as well as the following foods:-

IRON (Blood) FOODS

Beets	Rye	Yellow Corn
Lettuce	Asparagus	Pears
Spinach	Cherries	All Berries
Lentils	Peaches	Apples, Grapes
Tomatoes	Raisins	Green Beans
Peas	Dates	Raw Egg Yolk
Onions	Currants	Whole Wheat
Carrots	Cucumbers	Whole Barley
Prunes	All Nuts	Unpolished Rice
	Red Cabbage	

5. CHLORINE

Chlorine reduces fat tissues, cleanses the body, purifies the blood. Deficiency of Chlorine causes catarrh, pyorrhea, ulcers, body odors, skin eruptions, poor liver, kidney affections and obesity. When reducing weight take very little water or other fluids, or watery fruits and vegetables.

CHLORINE (Purifying) FOODS

Goat's Milk	Fish	Oranges
Goat's Cheese	All Greens	Limes
Organic Salt	All Melons	All Berries
Tomatoes	Carrots	RoquefortCheese
Radishes	Lemons	Raw Egg Yolk
Lettuce	Grapefruit	Lentils
Coconut	Cucumbers	Asparagus
Spinach		Raw Cabbage

6. SODIUM

Sodium keeps the body tissues pliable, gives one grace, speed, suppleness, prevents hardening of the arteries and stiffening of the joints. Sodium neutralizes acids of the blood and stomach, therefore is valuable in rheumatism, catarrh, high blood pressure, acidosis, gastric affections, etc.

SODIUM (Anti-acid) FOODS

Apples	Carrots	Gooseberries
Lentils	Cucumbers	Steel-cut Oats
Figs	Dates	Strawberries
Honey	Prunes	Raw Turnips
Spinach	Nuts	Peaches

Beets	String Beans Celery	Organic Salt

7. SILICON

Silicon is an integral part of the hair, skin and nails. Eat plenty of Silicon foods to improve the growth and texture of these organs. All very valuable for the nervous system and as a system tonic.

SILICON (Hair and Skin) FOODS

Cucumbers	Spinach	Cabbage
Rye	Barley	Oats
Nuts	Endive	Unpolished Rice
Cherries	Asparagus	Peaches
Whole Wheat	Apples	Dates
Beechnuts	Egg Yolk	Goat's Milk
Carrots	Peas	Strawberries
Figs	Grapes	Gooseberries

8. MAGNESIUM

Magnesium is the nerve tissue building element, also valuable for weak eyes and nervous affections. Persons who find relaxation difficult, are tensed, nervous, anxious, should drink plenty of grapefruit juice, unsweetened, during the day, and especially before retiring to relax the nerves.

The extracts of celery are also exceedingly valuable for the nerves. Steep this in the way you make tea, and drink it hot before retiring as well as with the meals.

MAGNESIUM (Nerve) FOODS

Raw Egg Yolk	Dates	Prunes
Coconut	Corn	Limes
Grapes	Cherries	Goat's Milk
Oats	Apples	Chestnuts
Peas	Lemons	Rye
Spinach	Beechnuts	Gooseberries
Almonds	Barley	Oranges
Walnuts	Peaches	Grapefruit

9. FLUORINE

Use a heavy fluorine diet in consumption, syphilis, skin diseases, gland and vein enlargements, anaemia, ulcers, open sores.

FLUORINE (Healing) FOODS

Egg Yolks	Goat's Milk	Cod Liver Oil
Spinach	Beets	Water Cress
Dates	Cauliflower	Steel-cut Oats
Cabbage	Swiss Cheese	Roquefort Cheese
Garlic	Sauerkraut	Brussels Sprouts
	All Fish	

10. IODINE

Indispensable to the endocrine glands for normal function. Iodine prevents goitre and in many cases cures it. This element is responsible for the pigmentation of the skin and hair. Everybody needs iodine in abundance to preserve the qualities of youth. Iodine balances the body's weight, destroys toxins in the system, burns up dead cells and tissues, and is splendid as a brain stimulant.

IODINE (Gland) FOODS

Japanese Kelp	Tomatoes	Oysters
Cod Liver Oil	Pineapple	Peas
Grapes (green)	Pears	All Fish
Strawberries	Mushrooms	Garlic
Lettuce	Irish Moss	Dulse
Raw Egg Yolk (in orange juice)		Onions
Skin of Baked Potato		

11. POTASSIUM

This is the laxative element, also gives energy to the heart, induces sleep, and is a general tonic for the whole body. Persons with sluggish intestines should eat plenty of potassium foods.

POTASSIUM (Laxative) FOODS

Cereals	Asparagus	Prunes
Bran	Oats	Mint
Lentils	Dates	Spinach
Apples	Figs	Carrots
Dandelion	Endive	Blackberries
Peas	Herbs & Teas	Whole Wheat
Lettuce	Nuts	Dried Olives
Potato Skin	Coconut	Cress

12. MANGANESE

Indispensable to brain and nerves, enabling the brain fibres to connect, thus promoting co-ordinating of thought and purpose. Valuable for the eyes and all nerve afflictions. Stammering, erratic judgment, worry, mental depression and other disturbing devitalizing conditions are often traced to lack of Manganese.

MANGANESE (Tonic) FOODS

Grapefruit	Endive	Honey
Pinon Nuts	Parsley	Raw Egg Yolk
Celery	Cress	Wintergreen
Walnuts	Almonds	Peppermint

Do not make the mistake of eating ONLY the foods specified for certain conditions.

Endeavor to get a wide variety of other foods with those indicated. Never use the same food every day, as this causes skin affections. There are many valuable foods which we have not listed here, but the foregoing are the richest in FOOD SALTS.

FLESH BUILDING FOODS

Olive Oil	Sweet Potatoes	Steel cut Oats
Cod Liver Oil	Brown Sugar	Lentils
Butter	Maple Sugar	Sweet Corn
Cream	Honey	Fruit Cake
Milk	Maple Syrup	Whole Wheat
Buttermilk	Malted Nuts	Sweet Berries
Rich Cheese	Prunes	Cherries
Eggs	All Nuts	Oranges
Malted Milk	Olives	Dates

Note:- Do not over eat. Take nourishment only when hungry and eat plenty of other natural foods, such as green salads, fresh fruits, berries, nuts and dairy products. Drink plenty of water. You may try mixing half a glass of orange juice, half glass of cream, one raw egg yolk, and honey to sweeten. Take each day with meals or between meals. It is a good idea to eat more frequently but in smaller amounts. Steel-cut Oats are valuable if soaked overnight in cream and eaten with honey or dates the following morning. Raw cracked wheat may be used the same way.

FLESH REDUCING FOODS

Lemons	Lettuce	Vegetable Soup
Salt Fish	Celery	Green Salads
Limes	Spinach	Raw Cabbage
Grapefruit	All Greens	Iodine Foods
Tomatoes	Salty Foods	Calcium Foods
All Melons	All Berries	Chlorine Foods

Note:- Take the juice of half a lemon several times a day without sweetening, between meals and before retiring. Use water and liquids sparingly. Avoid congestion of the vital organs, and develop the deep breathing habit. Exercise may also be necessary to procure complete results, but determine to follow instructions for at least six weeks and results are bound to reward you. Other foods should be used, but sparingly. Remember, also, the mental attitude has a great deal to do with the condition of one's weight. Therefore, endeavor always to keep the mind free of distress, as this condition may produce excessive weight or just the opposite. The proper amount to reduce is from two to three pounds a week, therefore do not reduce too quickly, as it is difficult to maintain results after they are effected.

On the following page is a list of certain specific FOODS Which may be used in the conditions for which they are indicated. This list has been prepared after exhaustive research work in Food Chemistry and has been proven to be exceedingly valuable.

NATURE'S MEDICINES

ALMONDS-Useful in cases of dysentery, and affections of the urinary organs; excellent for muscles, brain and nerves. All nuts, being a strong food, should not be eaten late in the day, or between meals, but should be taken with plenty of fresh fruit only as a complete meal.

APPLES- "The King of Fruits." Good for hot and bilious constitutions. All who suffer with acidity, gout, jaundice, indigestion, sluggish liver, nervousness, skin eruptions and allied troubles find them beneficial. They promote sound and restful sleep.

APRICOTS, PEACHES, NECTARINES-Very good for those suffering with worms and consumption.

ARTICHOKES - Very useful in cases of dropsy and jaundice.

ASPARAGUS- Easily digested; exerts a gentle, stimulating action, inducing perspiration, cleansing lungs and kidneys; excellent in asthma, consumption and Bright's disease.

BEETS-Promote digestion, are good for affections of brain, eyes, jaundice, erysipelas, and all skin diseases. Leaves to be used like spinach.
BEET JUICE-Greatest of all blood tonics. Grind the raw beets through a meat chopper, then press out the juice. Juice of half a lemon may be added to each glass of beet juice. Drink one glass daily. Should beets be dry, the pulp may be steeped slowly and the extracts taken.
BLACKBERRIES - Very good in diarrhea, dysentery, fevers, kidney diseases.
CABBAGE - Antiscorbutic; good for afflictions of the eyes, asthma, consumption, gout, scurvy; in building enamel of the teeth, nails and hair.
CARROTS - Good in cases of asthma, nervousness and dropsy; beautify the complexion and hair.
CAULIFLOWER-See cabbage.
CELERY-Excellent for brain fag, neuralgia, rheumatism, scrofula, gout, sciatica, obstruction of the liver and kidneys.
CHERRIES - The black are good for stone and gravel; red for removing tough phlegm humors.
COCONUT - An excellent food; the fresh nut ground and mixed with its own milk, will expel tapeworms; the milk, used in all cases of fever and exhaustion.
CRANBERRIES - Good for cancer, liver

troubles, bile, scurvy, erysipelas; makes an excellent drink in asthma, fevers, etc.

CUCUMBERS - For acne, ulcers of bladder, erysipelas and other inflammations, improves complexion.

CURRANTS - (black) Form one of the most useful fever beverages; good for coughs, colds, sore mouth and throat.

CURRANTS - (red or white) See Cranberries.

DANDELION - Good for ague, consumption, dyspepsia, dropsy, gravel, liver and kidney troubles. The root makes an excellent drink - good blood food.

DATES - An excellent food; good for those with poor circulation, gives heat to the body.

ELDERBERRIES - Excellent for sore throat, coughs, colds, etc.

ENDIVE - Good for liver, kidney or heart trouble, dimness of sight, for fevers, scurvy, jaundice.

FIGS - An excellent food; invaluable also for cancer, dropsy, scurvy, etc.

FILBERTS - Good for those who follow hard outdoor labor.

GARLIC - A stimulant, and good for asthma, dropsy, fevers, hysteria, worms, high blood pressure, rheumatism.

GOOSEBERRIES - Good for liver and stomach affections.

GRAPES - "The Queen of Fruits." Rich in chlorine, glucose, iron, lime, magnesium, phosphoric acid, potash, silicic soda, sulphuric acid, tartaric acid, etc. Excellent for blood building, good for consumption, fevers, dyspepsia, liver and kidney complaints, piles, etc.

GRAPEFRUIT - Greatest of all liver tonics. Slice it skin and all, then soak over night in one pint of water. Drink the extracts upon arising, to alternate with lemon-rich in organic quinine, it is recommended for fevers, headaches, biliousness, poor complexion, halitosis, high blood pressure, sluggish intestines. Splendid nerve tonic.

HONEY - A concentrated food, easy of assimilation, imparts warmth and energy. Many uses as remedial agent, excellent in throat and lung affection and in diseases of bladder and kidneys. A laxative and sedative.

LEMONS - Greatest of all blood purifying medicines. The juice from half a lemon, taken upon arising in the morning to - cleanse the stomach, purify the breath, stimulate the liver, strengthen the action of the bowels, purify the blood and tone up the entire system. Good for biliousness, dyspepsia, low fevers, gout, rheumatism, scurvy, liver and kidney troubles. A powerful antiscorbutic.

LETTUCE - Contains much iron and is therefore good for anaemic persons; recommended in insomnia, irritation of stomach, dyspepsia, etc.

MELONS - Excellent kidney cleanser.
MINT - Good for bowel complaints, affections of the heart, smallpox, etc.
ONIONS - Good for blood; cleanse whole system; good for insomnia, nervousness, coughs, etc.
ORANGES - Good for bronchitis, asthma, liver and heart troubles, for toning up the whole system and purifying the blood.
PARSLEY - One of the greatest kidney and bladder remedies in Nature's Botanical Garden. This should be bruised first, then steeped in hot water (not boiling) for half an hour. One bunch may be used to one quart of water. Drink from 2 to 6 glasses daily. An excellent remedy for dropsy, gravel, liver troubles, syphilitic affections and purifying the blood.
PARSNIPS - Good for dyspeptics.
PEARS - An excellent laxative when soft and ripe.
PEAS - Are good for hypochondria.
PINEAPPLE - An excellent remedy for diphtheria, sore throat, etc.
POMEGRANATES - Good for sore throat, lung complaints, hemorrhages, tapeworms, etc.
POTATOES - Excellent stomach cleanser.
QUINCES - and honey for Laxative. Good in all stomach troubles, will stop vomiting.
RADISHES - Furnish excellent treatment for gallstones.

RAISINS - Furnish sugar in purest and most concrete form. A fine heat and energy food.
RASPBERRIES - Good in cholera, sore throat, fevers, etc.
RHUBARB - Nature's most wholesome substitute for vinegar. A fine tonic and eliminator; good for cancer.
SAGE - Valuable in lung complaints, piles, rheumatism, and checking flatulency (gas).
SPINACH - Good in anaemia, heart disease, piles, stomach and kidney trouble.
STRAWBERRIES - Good for acne, gout, ringworm. Good outward application for cure of old wounds, ulcers, sore eyes and inflamed parts.
TOMATOES - Beneficial in dyspepsia, inflammations; good kidney and liver remedy.
TURNIPS - Excellent appetizer, good for ulcers of bladder; skin diseases and bone material.
WALNUTS - Pounded with honey are good for quinsy and sore throat.
WATERCRESS - Powerful blood cleanser, good for liver, kidneys, anemia, scurvy, etc. Useful in disorders of brain and bladder.
WHEAT MEAL - Made into a jelly and mixed with honey, is good for all lung troubles, for gout, hoarseness, rheumatism, etc. Good for chilblains, ulcers and boils, applied externally.

Remember CORRECT EATING is the important feature in effecting cures.

Progressive physicians are universally agreed on this. However, other elements are necessarily important. Such natural curative remedies as FRESH AIR, PURE WATER, APPROPRIATE EXERCISE, RELAXATION, SUNSHINE, PROPER BATHING, POSITIVE MENTAL ATTITUDE, etc., have an integral part to play in organizing HEALTH EQUILIBRIUM ON THE HUMAN BODY.

It is impossible to prescribe an exact diet for a nation to follow. Each individual is a law unto himself in this respect. However, the foregoing information should supply one with sufficient knowledge of FOOD CHEMISTRY to select a satisfactory diet to meet his individual requirements. Remember FOOD will cure or kill, according to its selection and use. Ninety-five percent of our diseases are caused from dietetic errors, therefore eliminate the errors. With a sufficient supply of other natural curative elements-such as Fresh Air, Sunshine, Relaxation, Appropriate Exercise, Fresh Water, Internal and External Cleanliness, and healthy Mental Attitude, and Nature will invariably provide the CURE - Excepting in very advanced stages of chronic or acute disease.

Persons who have acquired the habit of over-eating will do well to change their diet to more satisfying natural foods. One does not "overeat" of fruit, berries and vegetables, (which are man's natural foods), but when unnatural foods such as fried eggs, fried meat, fried potatoes, fried ham, fried bread, greasy pastry, rich cake, white flour products, corn starch products, syrups, cane sugar, candy, coffee mixed with cream, etc., are consumed even in moderate amounts, these invariable cause distress, and thereby so depress or alter the chemistry of the blood that other DISEASES result. Healers see fit to designate each separate symptom of DISEASE with a different name; this confuses one not acquainted with the processes of the body chemistry, whereas, these are but symptoms of one principal cause.

PART II

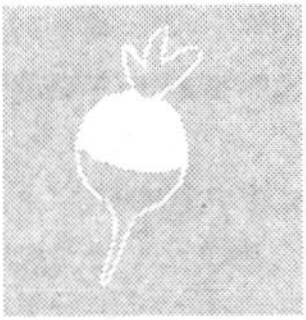

How to diet with Color

This, the latest scientific treatise on the subject of Color in Food, is based on the findings of the world's leading Color-Scientists over a period of fifty years.

Much of the information contained herein is taken from the laboratory experiments of Dr. J. E. Simons, the Color-Scientist of San Francisco, California, and includes twenty-five years of painstaking research for the benefit of humanity.

This work is verified by the International Society of Chromatologists of which Dr.

Simons is a member, and also by such authorities as Dr. Geiger, of the Department of Public Health of San Francisco, and Dr. Royal S. Copeland, Senator from New York State (deceased).

This is the identical system now in use in many of the large institutions of Germany, France and Italy, and also in California, at the Burbank Sanitarium.

Color indicates the mineral in the food, and when this absolutely scientific and easy method is followed, the weight will be normal, the breath and blood pressure will be natural, and all of the bodily functions will be working smoothly and harmoniously.

By balancing the Color of your food, you automatically balance the Vitamins, the Calories, and the Minerals, and 90% of the difficulty is eliminated.

Put yourself in harmony with true science and nature, and you will be a healthy, happy, successful human being.

Dieting with Color

Vibration is Life: That is one of the basic laws of the Universe. The sun is the source of the highest and most intense vibration in our physical world. Therefore, it logically follows that Sun is the source of the physical life of every living-thing on our planet.

Contrary to the general opinion, the Sun gives off no light or heat, only that intense vibration, which is only interpreted in terms of Light and Color by the Human Brain. Consequently, in order to be accurate and scientific, we must always work in terms of vibration, as that is the fundamental law of force which is interpreted by the human brain as Light, Color and Sound, according to the RATE of vibration.

When sunlight or white light, contacts any living organism all of the minerals necessary to growth and propagation are extracted from the sunlight, and the portion which is not needed is reflected. Man sees this reflected Color which has been thrown off by the plant, vegetable or fruit, and he says it is a certain Color. Actually it has absorbed all the colors in the sunlight, *except* the one he sees.

Science has now proven beyond the shadow of doubt, by the most delicate instruments ever invented, that Color always indicates mineral, whether it be Planet, plant, animal or human.

We now have instruments so sensitive that the light of a Planet can be passed through a prism and broken up into the several Colors of the Solar Spectrum. These colors each indicate a different mineral, and by the width of the bands of the separate colors, the proportion of the minerals on that

Planet can be seen and the Planet Weighed, Wonderful, isn't it?

So you see, my friends, that Color was given us, not merely to look pretty, but as an accurate, scientific guide to living. Wise is the man or woman who has the insight intuition and broadness of mind, to realize the possibilities of this new age of Color, and harmonize themselves with it. The field of vibration and its thousand and one uses, offers an absolutely limitless field of profit and interest to the discerning person who will grasp the opportunity, NOW!

Science has adopted the Angstrom Unit as the yardstick with which to measure Color vibrations. This Unit of Color measurement corresponds to the Watt of Electricity, and is simply an easy way of the three million or more tints which we derive from the three primary Colors, Red, Blue and Yellow.

We use six Colors instead of the seven in the Solarspectrum, and in addition, Black, White and Gray, as follows:-

Red	1500 Angstrom Units
Orange	1000 Angstrom Units
Yellow	500 Angstrom Units
	Faster than White Light.
Green	500 Angstrom Units
Blue	1000 Angstrom Units
Violet	1500 Angstrom Units
	Slower than White Light.

Black	1800 Angstrom units *Negative*
White	250 Angstrom Units *Influential*
Gray	300 Angstrom Units *Neutral*
Brown	1000 Angstrom Units *Basic*

There are several ways in which the Colors may be used in Diet. One is to eat all foods of one Color, each day (6 Basic Colors). Another is to use as many Colors as you wish at each meal, and balance them mathematically. Another is to eat foods of a certain Color each meal, which would complete the six basic colors every two days. Black, Brown, Gray and White are not necessary as they are contained in the first six colors.

So beneficial is this method, that persons who were slowly starving on the foods recommended by leading diet specialists, were, by having the same diet properly balanced according to Color, enabled to thrive and gain as much as twenty pounds in three months.

If you are overweight, this method will also enable you to reduce normally and in harmony with Nature. When we work with nature, instead of against her, she will bring about a balance, mentally, Emotionally and Physically.

Below we have a large variety of foods at one meal, giving the method of balancing according to Color. This can be done by ordinary arithmetic in five minutes. Always consider the Color of the food as it is served at the table.

Tomatoes, Beets- Red- 1500	2 Parts
Oranges - Orange - 1000	3 Parts
Sweet Potatoes, Carrots - Yellow	6 Parts
500 L. C. M. - 3000	
Lettuce, Spinach, Green Olives	6 Parts
Green - 500	
Coffee or Postum - Brown - 1000	3 Parts
Buttermilk, Celery - White - 250	12 Parts
Blueberries - Blue -1000	3 Parts

3000 is simply the Least Common Multiple, or the smallest number which will contain all of the others.

In this way we have quickly and easily balanced many foods so that they are equal in force or effect and the results will always be beneficial.

If several Colors are used at each meal, be sure that in the course of a day or two, you use foods of all the six basic colors, as a lack of one or more over a period of time will spoil the beneficial effect.

This is the only possible way aside from a chemical analysis, that diet can be balanced with anything even approaching accuracy.

Below will be found a chart which will guide you in your choice of minerals according to Color, and the effect of each mineral on the body.

SULPHUR (Pale Yellow) - Kills germs, makes rich blood, tones the whole system. Intensifies emotion; clears the complexion.

IODINE (Bluish - black)- Controls gland and cell action. Eliminates poison; prevents goitre, helps wounds heal quickly. When heated gives off violet fumes.

POTASSIUM (Bluish color) - Invigorates; renders tissues elastic; helps to prevent hardening of arteries; stimulates liver. Produces alkalinity.

CALCIUM (White and grayish) - Counteracts acid, builds bone, hair and teeth, makes energy and endurance, aids digestion.

PHOSPHORUS (Soft yellow to red orange) - Brain and nerve builder, hair and bone builder; nourishes mental organs; stimulates passion; retards old age.

IRON (Orange, rust, blood and red color) - Supplies energy and vitality; absorbs oxygen; enriches blood Rich blood prevents contagion.

MANGANESE (Reddish gray) - Builds tissue resistance; strengthens sense and thought nerves.

CHLORINE (Green) - Expels waste, freshens, cleanses and purifies the system.
MAGNESIUM (White) - Refreshes brain and nerves.
SODIUM (Silver white - gray white) - Checks digestive fermentation; good digestive aid and blood purifier.
FLUORINE (Pale green) - Skin beautifier and disease resistor.
SILICON (Dull brown) - Stability, reserve, ability to stand strain. Muscle and tissue builder.
CARBON (Coal black to white) - Energy and heat producer, when combined with fats and oils.
Oxygen, Hydrogen, Nitrogen (Water-white, gaseous).

When physical disease becomes acute through neglect, certain minerals must be introduced into the system in large quantities in order to restore the balance. This necessitates a temporary unbalanced diet until a condition of ease or balance is restored. When an acute condition becomes serious, so that the layman is unable to handle the situation, a skilled Dietician or Natural Practitioner should be called in before it is too late. If the directions contained in this and my other charts on the subject of Food and Color are conscientiously followed, you will rarely, if ever, need to consult a practitioner of any kind.

Below are the percentages of the minerals necessary to maintain a normal, healthy, and balanced body:-

Oxygen.	65%
Carbon.	18%
Hydrogen.	10%
Nitrogen	3%
	96%

Organic Mineral Salts

Calcium	1.50%
Phosphorus	1.00%
Potassium	0.35%
Sulphur	0.25%
Sodium	0.15%
Magnesium	0.05%
Iron	0.004%
Iodine	0.0004%
Chlorine	0.85%
Fluorine	Trace
Silicon	Trace
Manganese	Trace
	3.38904%

On the following page, you will find a variety of foods arranged according to Alkalinity and Acidity. By eating 80%

Alkaline foods, the Chemistry of the body will be enabled to maintain its balance, and health will be continuous.

FOODS HAVING BASIC REACTIONS IN THE BODY

(Use 80%)

MILDLY ALKALINE FOODS

FRUITS

Pears	Bananas	Oranges
		Peaches
Plums	Coconuts	Apricots
Watermelons	Lemons	Cherries
Grapejuice	Pineapples	Grapes
Apples	Raspberries	Muskmelons
	Currants	

MISCELLANEOUS

Milk

VEGETABLES

Cauliflower	Radishes	Rhubarb
Onions	Tomato juice	Turnips
Pumpkin	Cucumbers	Cabbage
Asparagus	Lettuce	Mushrooms
String Beans	Potatoes	Green Peas
Sweet Potatoes		Tomatoes

MODERATELY ALKALINE FOODS

FRUITS

Figs	Dates	

VEGETABLES

Fresh Beans	Beets	Parsnips
Watercress		Carrots

MISCELLANEOUS

Chestnuts

HIGHLY ALKALINE FOODS

FRUITS

Olives	Dried Prunes	Raisins

VEGETABLES

Dry Beans	Kale	Soy Beans
Chard	Lima Beans	Turnip Greens
	Spinach	

MISCELLANEOUS

Almonds	Molasses

NEUTRAL FOODS

Butter	Lard	Sugar
Cornstarch	Cream	Tapioca

FOODS HAVING ACID REACTIONS IN THE BODY

(Use 20%)

Least Acid Forming Foods

MEAT AND FISH

Bacon	Salmon	Trout
	Perch	

CEREAL PRODUCTS

Green Corn	Dried Sw. Corn	Crackers

MISCELLANEOUS

Egg White	Peanuts	Lentils

MODERATELY ACID FORMING FOODS

MEAT AND FISH

Beef Ribs	Canned Salmon	Pork
Sardines	Frog	Pike
Ham	Halibut	

CEREAL PRODUCTS

Whole Wheat Bread	Barley	White Breakfast Food
	Rice	

MISCELLANEOUS

Walnuts	Whole Egg	Cheese

VERY ACID FORMING FOODS

MEAT AND FISH

Beef	Rabbit	Haddock
Chicken	Veal	Oysters
	Venison	

CEREAL PRODUCTS

Oatmeal	Spaghetti	Macaroni

MISCELLANEOUS

Egg Yolk

Other Titles in this Series
BY PILGRIMS PUBLISHING

Herb Garden .... *Helen Lyman*

Sleep & Samadhi .... *Sister Devamata*

What is Maya? .... *Sister Devamata*

How To Get Your Winning Number .... *Lewis de Clairemont*

The Twelve Healers .... *Edward Bach*

The Science Of The Aura .... *S.G.J Ouseley*

Psychoanalysing The Twelve Zodiacal Types ...... *Manly P. Hall*

The Therapeutic Value of Music .... *Manly P. Hall*

Astrology and Reincarnation .... *Manly P.Hall*

The Noble Eightfold Path .... *Manly P.Hall*

The Symbolism Of The Tarot .... *P.D. Ouspensky*

How To Select A Guru? .... *Ramamurti S. Mishra*

Buddhism & Lamaism .... *J.E. Ellam*

The Mysticism Of Sound .... *Inayat Khan*